LOVE/RESISTANCE /REBELLION

A collection of poetry

P M HILL

chipmunkapublishing
the mental health publisher

P M HILL

All rights reserved, no part of this publication may be reproduced by any means, electronic, mechanical photocopying, documentary, film or in any other format without prior written permission of the publisher.

> Published by
> Chipmunkapublishing
> United Kingdom

http://www.chipmunkapublishing.com

Copyright © 2020 P M Hill

ISBN   978-1-78382-5288

TELL HIM

If you see him
Tell him
I'm sorry
For that sibling rivalry
Turned ugly

If you see him
Tell him

He is amazing
Has a "heart of gold"

If you see him

My friend, confidante and
Soulmate

Tell him
My achievements
Are nothing without him

And ask him

To reveal the contents of
That unsent letter when
I was psychotic

Helpless
And estranged from home,

Tell, tell and tell him again

He is
Under-valued by a world

Hung up on individual productivity
Under-valuing others like him
Thank him for being him
That is enough and always will be

From me
Who messed up time and again

Didn't understand and never will

Fully

How much he helped me

Through that journey
From those dark, dark ethical spaces
How lonely that would've been
After my wife died

LOVE/RESISTANCE/REBELLION

Tell him

I never acknowledged
Let alone help him process
The oppression, grief and mutual loss

If you see him
Tell him he is loved

My world would've been so much poorer

Without him

SORRY MUM

Took me on
At that time
Me and my brother
Sacrificed
Everything
You said

Four walls for your
Company
Endless chores
Said you loved me
Did not
Believe you

You told me off
Looking at me with disgust
Said I could play
In that square-metre
If there was no mess
Said I could cry
But for the right things

So, mum
After nearly fifty years
I'm sorry

LOVE/RESISTANCE/REBELLION

For my imperfections, my moody silences
I was the best
I could be

But
You tell the neighbours
About your pride
Of two grown up brothers
My photographic memory
My success at school
Never once sharing
That in my ear-space

I never told you
About the bus
I almost threw myself
Under at the age of twelve

Always looking for your
Disappointed look
That hectoring voice
That said you cared
But received with
Contempt

I had seen you cry
When saying farewell

On that
Campus in Leicester
And I didn't understand

Yet
You ventured on a
Thousand-mile trip

To be there in my moment of grief
That hug that said
I love you
And I believed it
And I understood

But mum
I lived to see
Those traumas through
To love myself
By the grace of God, I do.

Sorry we didn't see
Eye to eye

And yes, I stopped

Blaming you

LOVE/RESISTANCE/REBELLION

For my inadequacy

No longer the victim
I thought I was
Re-invented through
Communion with
The true vine

You led me to water
But you could break
My Spirit
Instead
Led to the
Altar of bread and wine

Re-nurtured

Re-born

Re-made

THE CONFINED SPACE

In that space
Dare I stray
Too far left or right
Or make much mess
Dare I utter a dis-chorded note
Or mutter or cry

On the back-burner
I must be

So that

The authority figures can
De-cry

So that

I am not a hindrance

But

Things are far from okay
And I want to stray
Outside that square-metre

Of space

LOVE/RESISTANCE/REBELLION

Or make
A meaningful cry

I wanted to encounter
The messiness of life

Even if it causes me strife,

But there I was in this square-metre of space

From which I cannot stray

Until the day

When that space implodes

A tiny a corpse in

Lifeless diminutive shell

And I am zombified

Within that chemical hell

My face, mask-like and drawn

Until the medication

Is fine tuned to a lesser dawn

FORGIVEN

Remembering the time
You opened up to me about

The nature of that gilded cage
People said your wings had been
Clipped as well

You checked and checked again so
Like you always
Did and that routine that
Said that important chores
Done on auto-pilot

We knew where we were and
At what time and what we would
Eat on what day

You opened up
To tell me you had been
Tempted to leave

That cage but
For your children you
Would have done so
You told us of four
Walls that almost drove you

Insane

You checked out
For shopping trips to town but
You never felt you could leave
Three children behind
To fend for themselves
Without you

But

Without you

Things could have been
Worse and in the end, you felt it
Was better that you
Made the sacrifice kept
Silent and made do

You had experienced the
Brutality of an upbringing in
War and the
Austerity that followed

Trauma and humiliation were
Your soul-mates then

LOVE/RESISTANCE/REBELLION

But
You couldn't help pass down those
Soulmates and bedfellows to your
Own children
Like a copper-plated
Semi-conductor

And my troubled conscience
Can finally understand
Your generation and
Their struggle to communicate
Love

I know you made up for lost time
Telling us you
Loved us at
Those family
gatherings

I fear you still even now

But
Knowing, wanted the best for
Your three children and
Your grand-children

I can forgive with a glad and
Thankful heart

SONNET

This is the sonnet
For the woman that
Glanced at me
And gave me
That knowing
Smile

For the woman whose
Gaze held my own for
Those still precious
Seconds

For the person who
Dared to enter my world
However fleetingly, momentarily
And superficially
This is for you

You captured
In those short still
Seconds

The yearning, the vulnerability,
The demeanour,
That only you could
And broke down my-

Defenses

So, for now I yearn for
Another fleeting look
That only you can give
So that my splintered
Wounded and experienced
Heart can be full
Overflowing
And dare I say it mended

This is a sonnet for you

THE GILDED CAGE.

Those wings were clipped
At 19

The wedding-cake cut
Her fate sealed

Those four walls were built
At 23
Their mortgage brokered
Her cards dealt

Those children were born
At 24
Fostered
Till 18
The maximum sentence

Those children came of age at 41.
Their sentence served
The cage open

That open door
At 47
The fledglings had flown
Her wings were unfurled

With no-where to fly to

EMOTIONAL GOLDFISH

Emotional goldfish
In a pond
Wrapped in themselves
Their default-position

Reacting

Others, the rational type
open minded
Think 10 steps ahead
Making that journey
From heart to head

Thinking

Other aquatic types
in the ocean
Forget the mess of the past
Their default-position
Repeat mistakes
Break the bonds with those
they love
Cannot be saved
from themselves

Strangling, suffocating

Manipulating and controlling
They destroy
And are helpless

Those insightful
Oriental fish
in goldfish bowls
Remember their-
Fortunate past

And
Remain there

The bowl is in the ocean
But never venture out

Pleased to be
In that familiar zone
Who don't understand the other fish
And their messiness

They are puzzled

There are those who start in
The pond as goldfish
And journey from
The pond
Who still sometimes

Are unable to help themselves
They learn and re-learn from
The messiness of the past

They are hopeful

But

Every time they re-learn, the longer
They breath without
replenishment they
become bigger fish
And the pond
Grows bigger as their
Encounters grow in number

They are beacons

Better, to grow in the pond
And to venture out
Better to make mistakes in
A cycle of almost never-
ending learning and re-learning
Than to stay in the bowl
And lose touch

Those that never reach out
The pond or river
Cannot be saved
They become less relevant

One day
Left behind on the shore
They struggle to breath and are a warning to
The other puzzled fish

WOODCOCK STREET BREAKDOWN

There were times
When I doubted myself in that battery-farm
They called the office

Granted that square-metre of space
to breath in that
Suffocation

Battered by the visits
To assess those needs
I took solace in those times
And that place where I could
Breath in that public house

Swayed one way then the other
By that Carer, that Nurse, that Manager

And I could not find
My own still voice of calm
Explaining other people's
Decisions, mistakes and
Rulings

I surrendered
Taking the blame that wasn't mine to own

And drowning in that sea of drink

I let myself go

To surrender to the budget holder, the manager
And the proverbial candlestick maker
Losing myself but finding nothing in
Return.

I drowned to the depths of fate and I regressed
To a place where I struggle to breath and
Hemmed in on all sides

I implode in that place they call
Woodcock Street

LITTLE PINK RIDING HOOD

She's the petite kind
Who knows he's going out of his mind

About her, her face, freckles and false smiling

Entrapped by her own flirting nature

She too polite to say no
And too scared to say yes

Trapped by him
Who pursues her like the wolf
He's unrelenting, irrepressible, undaunted

What beautiful freckles you have

What charm you exude

What long flowing hair you caress

All the better to avoid you with

All the better to take the hint

All the better to take it on the chin

They lead the long merry dance

The pursuer and pursued

Month after month
Year after year

Until the parting
To their home-towns pending

Another academic year ending

Till he stops sending those e-mails, blogs and

Handwritten notes

Then

His house blows in
Then she reins him in
Young riding hood

Scared but intact

Young wolf like pursuer in grief
Broken, shattered, fractured

LOVE/RESISTANCE/REBELLION

To begin 30 years in mending
To regress
His mental health needs pending

BEFORE WELFARE

Aunt Dot proudly
Told a story of old
She had always been bold

We never had an NHS
And couldn't afford the GP

So, we made do

Bombs that fell
And shrapnel hit
No counselling for that

So, we made do

No nanny in the state
Welfare, Social Services or benefits

We kept calm and carried on

Pregnant out of wedlock
We took that baby in
Till he walked

Then they came back for him

LOVE/RESISTANCE/REBELLION

They made do

Ration cards that told you
What to eat and how much

We made do

I passed my eleven plus
Qualified for grammar school,

No bursary to go
I made do

UNCLE DAVIDS HISTORY LESSON

Uncle David recalled

Hindsight is a wonderful thing

In the history of earthlings

Like the ABBA song of old

History repeating itself

Mistakes of old, repeated in bold

Another story re-told

Hitler invading Russia

What a folly

Surely, he knew
It would end in retreat

And like Napoleon

In defeat

And in the great scheme of things

LOVE/RESISTANCE/REBELLION

No legacy

The victor writing
Their version

For posterity

ODE TO COVENTRY

Most of the Luftwaffe squadron
Reduced Coventry to a cauldron

As Bomber Harris did to Hamburg
Cologne and Dresden

The huge bomber formation
Carpet bombed the City
On their way in

And showed no mercy
As they bombed
From the other way on the run in

Four out of ten houses
Destroyed

Incendiary bombs
Employed

That bought down the Cathedral ceiling

Citizens of Coventry left reeling

In the morning just after dawn

LOVE/RESISTANCE/REBELLION

Tired haggard faces

Mask like and drawn

Trundled to work in shock

They kept calm and carried on
And on and on and on

Until a spring day in 1945

Many Londoners danced down the Mall

And in Leicester Square

And

The lesser known people in Coventry
Seemed like they had not got a care

But

Lest we forget

The suffering of Coventry, Cologne, Hamburg
And Dresden

And Lest we forget

The worst that was to come

As Hiroshima and Nagasaki
Succumbed

Their people numbed in shock

And out of rock

A new Cathedral built

And from the ruins of the Cathedral
Of old

The new building stood out bold

Reconciled and reconciling their bold

From nation to nation
To young and old

Past to present

LOVE/RESISTANCE/REBELLION

The visitors venture from the ruins of Good Friday

To the hope and peace of Easter Sunday

JOB LIKE LAMENT

I cry, cry, cry again

Wash, wash, wash
Cover and envelope me

Take, take, take

The very and complete
Essence of me

And

Remove the trace
I ever was, ever saw
Or ever knew

Still that ripple on the clear water
From the birthstone thrown
From the waters-edge

Destroy the time capsule

And consign everything to the deep

LOVE/RESISTANCE/REBELLION

Please, please, please
Let me be

Not that I should offend or
Curse or blaspheme the supreme being

Alas

There is no grace
In the tide of
Everlasting judgement

Love, love, love
If you want it

Should be free

So, get your dog
To lick your face with glee

And let
The inward tide

Wash, wash, wash
Over me

And let there be no longer any trace of me or anyone
Who could have been me

PRIDE

I am not proud
For even if it was a sin

I would love
To hold on those
Feelings for that
Moment
That said

The lad did well

And hold on to then very notion

That something about me
Even for the moment
Before the inevitable fall
I Could be deemed worthwhile

Alas
When those deeds
Of which I reflect on that
Were good

It is from those stormy places

And when the winds blow -

I have failed yet again

Longing to serve

But

From a default position
From which

I lack that possibility
Of transformation

The biggest lies, are the ones you tell yourself

And

In the spotlight of reality, I check and compare

I avoid the pain and the cost of what that would mean
And I am diminished, confused, deluded and out of touch

With the very notion I could have done well

GREAT GRANDPAS CAMPAIGN MEDALS

You're only
Someone in the Army

Great Grandpa said

So, he joined up
To get ahead

Born in Aston of Brummie stock
An Empire to defend

To uphold himself no end

General Kitchener
Assigned and conscripted

Liberation of Gordon in Khartoum

He enlisted

In vain for poor Gordon

But the Sudanese
Were defeated
Campaign medal with glee

He greeted

The Dutch settlers in South Africa took hold
and rebelled

Another campaign to unfold

Lady smith medal to uphold

Kitcheners poster-finger beckoning

He enlisted

Lying about his age and health

Emboldened

To the Army enlisted

Others were conscripted
Saying

You're a nobody unless
You join the army

Then you're a somebody

LOVE/RESISTANCE/REBELLION

In the trenches he fought

Another campaign medal he sought

Britain alone after Dunkirk
Again, he enlisted but was turned back and resisted.

Hop it mate and join the home guard they said

An honorary campaign medal instead

UNCLE PHIL

He's always been ill in the head
His odours we dread

A face that for years was mask-like and drawn

Then with medication changes overdue

He had a reserved awkward stare

Now it's as though he hasn't got a care

He's a decent bloke

With one-liner jokes

An agony uncle to all

When it comes to football, he knows

The score

And when he philosophizes – it's over your head

Just like the bad joke that you can't get out of your head

I wouldn't say he's over qualified

But with the letters after his name

He makes lesser mortals terrified

The eternal student

He studied while it was prudent
Then he was now told we've run out of courses
Back to the rat race

His interviews were ace

His new medication, getting him attention
To details

He now knows what his job entails

The knock on the door
Said that uncle Phil has arrived
Chancing to stay for coffee

Until a meal by his sister is contrived

LOVE AND SCHIZOPHRENIA

He doesn't know how it appears with schizophrenia

Knowing only his perception

His advances couldn't be clearer

And he finds her no-where near

The walk out to that winter sunshine

He finds out himself far out and is declined

His unwelcome size nines

Leave a clumsy mark on her heart

But let him take a look in the mirror

And get a few things clearer

Why is she not there?

Could she live in fear?

As those footsteps draw

Nearer

Seduction at its worst

He clearly failed to get there first

He feels his life is cursed

For even if he was the last person on earth

She would always give him a wide berth

Realizing now what he did then

Now in that chemical mayhem

Destroying himself because of what he couldn't get then

Testimonials

Philip Hill's powerful new collection does not flinch from exploring some of the key dilemmas that ultimately confront us all. What might it mean to acknowledge and recognize our pasts and ourselves; to forgive and to seek forgiveness; to be reconciled without deformity; and to discover – and speak boldly from – that place of integrity which is to be found in the deepest recesses of our being?

This is poetry to be spoken aloud and wondered at. It both consoles and challenges with its blend of tenderness, raw honesty and hard-won wisdom. Nourishment from a poet rich in maturity of voice and vision.

Fiona Breckenridge

Former PHD Student of English, Mentor, Friend

Poetry is a condensed and direct form of words that speaks to a variety of human situations but it is especially suited to exploring the intricacies of human relationships, the accompanying emotions, the unspoken angst, and the unspeakable terror of rejection. Philip Hill, in these poems, has worked the magic of words, that combination of precise diction and euphony, that speak directly to the heart. I feel very honoured to have been asked to write a foreword for this collection of poetry. I have been moved and touched, and also changed. That, in the end is what poetry aims at.

Professor Femi Oybode

Professor of Psychiatry, University of Birmingham, Poet

Having known Philip since 2012, I consider him to be a friend, confidante, trustworthy soul-mate who I can relate to and understand, having empathy for his past experiences. I have become a person who has facilitated and fine-tuned his expression of his poetry, having felt no reason to alter the way he projects his thoughts onto paper. Despite the illness he has been diagnosed, Philip writes with such clarity, realism and with a huge understanding of humanity, expressing himself in an honest, sincere and insightful way to expose his most internal directional thoughts to the reader, connecting common human experiences on a deeper level.

Jemma Stone, Educationalist, Mentor, Friend, Typist, Proof-Reader

www.ingramcontent.com/pod-product-compliance
Ingram Content Group UK Ltd.
Pitfield, Milton Keynes, MK11 3LW, UK
UKHW041413180426
11947UKWH00007B/109